INTERMITTENT FASTING

HOW TO LOSE FAT FAST AND HEALTHY

JUSTINE YOUNG

CONTENTS

Introduction   v

1. What is Intermittent Fasting?   1
2. Health benefits of Intermittent Fasting   5
3. Pros and Cons of Different Intervals   9
4. Weight Loss and Intermittent Fasting   19
5. Beginner Mistakes on Intermittent Fasting   23
6. How to motivate yourself   29
7. Intermittent Fasting is not for everyone   33
8. Frequently asked questions   35

Afterword   39
Last Words   41
References   43

INTRODUCTION

Is there such a thing as easy weight loss? Well, if you are a pills person then you might say yes because to date there have been a lot of products on the market which promise no workout, only weight loss results in a matter of weeks. However, keep in mind that taking pills is still a hit or miss. It may or may not work for you, so technically, it's still not "easy".

I'm thinking that since you grabbed this book, you are not a pills person. Well, neither am I. Hence, this book is not about losing the excess pounds so that you will look good for the grand alumni homecoming, which will happen next month. This book isn't about a quick and easy weight loss scheme; it's about being healthy, more energized, and more in tune with your body. With intermittent fasting you can be all three: healthy, energized, and focused. No worries, though, because in the process of doing intermittent fasting, you will DEFINITELY lose weight.

In the dieting realm, there's no such thing as easy weight loss, so if you have the fascinating idea that intermittent fasting offers quick solutions to your extra weight problems, you might be a little disappointed.

Intermittent fasting isn't a one-time deal. It's something best done

INTRODUCTION

continually because the effects are outstanding. I must say that when it comes to the speed of results, intermittent fasting isn't lagging behind, but I don't want you to think that once you have gained the desired weight, you can discontinue the lifestyle. To get long-lasting results, you have to build a habit around it. But don't worry, I will show you how to achieve that, step by step. Even when you have a busy lifestyle.

Please note that this book is filled with honest facts. It is aimed to help you choose the right intermittent fasting interval for your lifestyle. If you want a diet system that will teach you to listen to your body and will leave you as much control as possible, intermittent fasting is the way to go.

In this book you will learn the following:

- The foundations of intermittent fasting and the science-backed reasons of why it works.
- Methods of motivating yourself while on the diet.
- The mistakes one often makes and how to avoid them (Clue: you should never, ever eat less than you need)
- Intermittent fasting do's and don'ts and why your body is literally the BOSS
- How you can lose weight just by skipping breakfast
- The different intervals and which is the best for you
- The pros and cons of different intervals
- Most frequently asked questions, like how much pounds can I possibly lose?
- And many more!

Before you begin your intermittent fasting journey, allow me to thank you for trusting me. I sincerely hope that you will have a lot of takeaways from this book. Go highlight statements and bookmark pages to your heart's content.

Happy reading!

1

WHAT IS INTERMITTENT FASTING?

Intermittent fasting, which we will frequently address as IF in this book, is not a new discovery. It has been performed by many people across different cultures even before it spread like wildfire via social media and various health and wellness websites. Believe me when I say that IF is one effective way to shed the unwanted pounds; still, before you can thoroughly follow through this very controlled diet system, you need to understand what it is and how it works fully.

Intermittent fasting is not starvation; it doesn't require you to resist the temptation of eating for hours on end. Because fasting sometimes becomes synonymous to starvation, it is commonly misinterpreted as the act of deliberate misery! Well, medical and nutrition science beg to disagree. According to experts, our body has two states when it comes to eating – the fasted and the fed. Fasted means the state when food doesn't enter our body and fed is our favorite part: eating. If we consider this meaning, it only follows that we do fasting EVERY DAY. We do it when we stop eating after lunch and when we "break our fast" in the morning. Sometimes we do it haphazardly to the point of starving ourselves, which of course, is not recommended.

Intermittent fasting adds control to the otherwise unsystematic diet. In this hype, you must cycle between the state of being fed and fasted for a specific duration or eating-window. For instance, the most popular time-frame is the 16:8 method wherein breakfast is skipped, your first meal is lunch at 12 o'clock, and you eat dinner at 8 in the evening. In this method, you are fasting for 16 hours – from after dinner to 12 in the afternoon. There are many more timeframes we will discuss later, but essentially IF is all about controlling *when* to eat.

While it helps to choose the kind of food, you'll eat, IF doesn't account for that. The only concern is when – not what. But then again, your body will thank you if you'll splurge on the healthy variety instead of the empty calories on the time that you actually choose to eat.

DOES IF WORK?

Considering the fact that civilization has benefited greatly from this method, consider intermittent fasting as a very effective way of not just losing the extra weight – it also keeps the body healthy.

Looking back to the days when home cooked meal was a luxury, our ancestors hunted for food. Since they didn't always have a deer around the corner to feast on, they fasted while searching for their next prey. Although they hadn't researched this method yet, they did benefit from it by giving their body enough time to fully process the food they had eaten, increasing their stamina and giving them the build of an effective hunter. In ancient Greece and Egypt, the physicians encouraged their patients to participate in a fasting period to prevent future diseases. In some religions, the members are asked to fast to reinforce their faith and validate self-control.

Now, though, fasting is seen in a new light what with all the new studies and testimonies from people who tried and become satisfied with this diet. According to Kris Gunnars, BSc, IF works by preventing you from consuming unnecessary calories. Unnecessary because we still have something in our body that we can use as energy (fats), so we don't really need to consume more. We will discuss more on the mechanism of IF when we get into the benefits, but for now, think about this:

When we fast, our body doesn't get the usual glucose dose which is easily processed as energy. Without it, our system will be forced to use the next available source: fats. Over a period of time, our body will be so accustomed to using fats that we will eventually lose the unwanted pounds. Fascinating, isn't it?

This is why intermittent fasting has taken the world by storm. With this book, I hope you will find the will and inspiration to try it out. Don't worry; we'll cover all bases to help you achieve your IF goal.

WHAT HAPPENS WHEN WE EAT?

Have you ever wondered – what happens to the food that we eat? Sure, it will be processed by our digestive system, but how do they really become useful to us?

Let's say you ate the ever-sinful, carb-rich pizza. From the mouth to the stomach, the pizza will be broken down into simple substances: the carbs will turn to glucose, the proteins into amino acids. These simpler versions of the molecules will be absorbed via the small intestine and taken into the bloodstream, which will deliver it to the liver where it will be processed further to be distributed to different parts of the body. When the molecules are not needed, the liver won't distribute them – it will simply keep it or transform it into another more "storable" substance for future use.

Well, you know that when we eat a lot, our body won't need all the contents of our food. Imagine eating a plateful of pasta and then eating 2 slices of cake for dessert only to sit for 3 hours in a meeting. You're on for a literal sugar-rush! The excess glucose (sugar) not needed by our cells will be stored in the liver as glycogen, but be wary, because our liver only has limited storage space. When that limited space is occupied, our liver will transform sugar into fats and store it to various parts of the body like the abdomen, arms, and thighs. The horror! You see, while glycogen stored in the liver is easily accessible, the distributed fats in the body are not; hence, it's difficult to lose them.

You can lose the extra pounds by reducing your food intake. This technique is geared toward using the fats already stored in the body rather than creating new fats. And this is where intermittent fasting enters the picture.

2.

HEALTH BENEFITS OF INTERMITTENT FASTING

Knowing that intermittent fasting is an age-old secret that a lot of people now are taking advantage of, I hope I can motivate you to do it; however, I know that you need more than just discovering what it is – as of this moment, you want to know the things you can get out of it. In this chapter, I'll try to be as scientific as I can without losing the touch of someone who was once a beginner in the IF realm. Let's get this started!

1. HELPS YOU BURN FAT AND LOSE WEIGHT

This is first on the list simply because losing weight is most likely the reason you picked up this book. Well, you'll be glad to know that two evidence-based facts connect INTERMITTENT FASTING to effective weight loss management.

First, because you are fasting, your normal caloric intake will decrease. Let's look at it this way: according to SFGate the highest daily caloric intake an active woman can have is 2,400. That figure is of course divided across all meals. If you take just 3 meals a day, you can have 800 calories in one seating! But what if you are following the Intermittent Fasting lifestyle, say the 16:8 method we covered earlier? 800 calories for lunch and another 800 for dinner - that's just 1600! So technically, following the IF routine means consuming less, giving your body enough chance to burn calories.

Next, intermittent fasting can boost your metabolic rate. Going through IF will evidently cause your insulin level to decrease, your growth hormones to increase, and add more norepinephrine in your system! All these will make your metabolism more active.

2. IF IS GOOD FOR YOUR BRAIN AND MAKES IT SHARPER

You see, it's not enough for us to have the body of our dreams, we also need to be sharp as tack because then we will definitely be admirable. According to Orsha Magyar, MSC, CHN, IF increases the BDNF or brain-derived neurotrophic factor, a protein that encourages the birth of neurons or brain cells. Additionally, BDNF reduces the degeneration of our brain cells. Because our neurons age less, the chances of having neurodegenerative diseases such as dementia and Alzheimer's will be slimmer.

The bottom line is this: new brain cells plus longer lasting neurons mean healthier cognitive function. Again, sharp as tack.

3. IF BENEFITS YOUR HEART HEALTH

Do you want to go from being admirable to irresistible real fast? Add a healthy heart to your fit body and sexy mind! As science would have it, intermittent fasting is a great lifestyle to maintain if you want to reduce the chances of developing heart diseases.

Did you know that in a study, it was observed that IF can help in the prevention and healing of ischemic heart injury which happens during myocardial infarction or stroke? With IF, the adiponectin serum level increases, promoting protection of the heart. Moreover, the participants who suffered from heart disease survived longer with IF!

Of course, with weight loss comes a ton of benefits for the heart.

Try browsing through the risk factors of coronary heart diseases, and you will find words like "obesity", "bigger waist circumference", "increased fat mass", "high blood pressure" and "too much bad cholesterol". With intermittent fasting, all the risk above factors can be eliminated or at least reduced.

There are many more reasons why Intermittent Fasting can be beneficial for your sweet heart, but in my humble opinion, you must be prepared to be bombarded by countless medical terms that sound way too unfamiliar. Still, if you chance upon the desire to look them up, here's a great collection of the studies: Cardioprotective Effects of Intermittent Fasting

4. IF LOWERS THE RISK OF TYPE 2 DIABETES

Earlier, you read that IF reduces the level of insulin. For those of you who are familiar with what insulin is, you might be as confused as I was when I was researching about IF. Insulin is a hormone meant to decrease the sugar in our blood. This is why diabetic people sometimes need to take insulin shots because if they don't, they risk experiencing hyperglycemia or abnormally high blood glucose levels. If this is the case, then how can intermittent fasting help lower the risk of Type 2 Diabetes when it decreases the insulin hormone? Wouldn't IF only promote high levels of blood sugar?

Let's all be enlightened by ascertaining what Type 2 Diabetes Mellitus (DM) is. According to the American Diabetes Association, Type 2 DM is the most common form of diabetes. It happens when the body *cannot properly use* insulin; a condition called insulin resistance. Because we cannot use the insulin, the glucose in our blood will remain high, giving the impression that there isn't enough insulin in the body. The pancreas (the organ the produces insulin) will compensate – releasing more of the said hormone. Over time, the pancreas won't be able to keep up.

Here's the game changer: with IF, insulin resistance can be reduced. In other words, going through the wheels of intermittent fasting will make our body use insulin more appropriately. So, yes – insulin is lowered, but whatever insulin our pancreas produces, our body can take advantage of it.

Another thing, insulin production is triggered by glucose levels in our blood. The higher the level is, the more our pancreas is commanded to release the hormone. Too much production, of course, tires our pancreas and problems can arise. With intermittent fasting, we are reducing our food intake. Thus we can worry less about having too much glucose.

And last but not least, medical studies state that one of the major risk factors of Type 2 DM is obesity. With IF, we can control our weight, so that's one less risk factor on our side.

5. INTERMITTENT FASTING CAN INCREASE LIFESPAN

Can IF increase our longevity? A Harvard study says so. In their study they used worms because they only live for about 2 weeks, giving them the chance to see the aging process real time. According to the Harvard researchers, we age in connection to our cells' reduced ability to use energy. And what part of our cell "produces" the energy? None other than our mitochondria – the powerhouse.

Our mitochondria have two states – the fused (youthful) and fragmented (aged). As we get older, they, of course, become fragmented and their ability to process energy declines leading to pronounced aging and vulnerability to age-related diseases. With intermittent fasting, the researchers found out that the worms actually maintained the fused mitochondria! Moreover, the youthful mitochondria promote lifespan by increasing fat metabolism.

What's in it for us? Abide by the IF routine, and you will enjoy life longer!

3

PROS AND CONS OF DIFFERENT INTERVALS

The best thing about intermittent fasting is you do it systematically while staying in complete control of the times you have to fast and be fed. In this chapter, we will lay down the choices including the benefits and possible disadvantages so that you may better choose your interval according to your lifestyle and personal preference.

Before we begin, a reminder that all these timeframes bear the benefits of intermittent fasting as listed in the previous section. From here on, the pros that we will mention are specifically about the interval.

THE 16:8 INTERVAL

The 16:8 method or interval is the most popular since according to many IF believers, it is the easiest. As mentioned earlier, in this method you need to fast for 16 hours and eat only in an eight-hour window. The previous example is the most common: you skip breakfast, eat your lunch at 12 pm and your dinner at 8 pm. Can you eat between lunch and dinner? Yes! That's why it's the *eating-window*. You can eat but preferably only small, healthy snacks. After dinner, it's fasting all the way until noon. You can change the time, though.

Meaning you can eat brunch at 10 am, eat dinner at 6 pm, and fast until it's 10 am again. Just as long as the concept of fasting for 16 hours and eating at a window of 8 hours remains, that's 16:8 IF.

The Pros

- The 16:8 method, according to many practitioners, is the easiest. All you need to do is skip breakfast, eat lunch, munch on a few healthy foods as snacks late in the afternoon, and then have your dinner. You fast while you are sleeping as you usually would.
- For people who are working early in the morning, this is a big advantage as skipping breakfast gives more room for other activities such as planning, preparing healthy lunch and snacks, or meditating.
- It is an inexpensive way to lose weight as you don't have to spend money on costly cereals, wheat bread, non-fat milk, and other items which you would only be buying to ensure that your breakfast is not loaded with too many carbs that can turn into fats.

The Cons

- If you like your breakfast, you might need to choose a different eating-window. Since it has been inculcated in our mind that "breakfast is the most important meal of the day", a lot of people may be having difficulty in letting it go.
- Self-control MUST be established to ensure that you won't compensate for the time when you are fasting. Others might feel "privileged" to eat more for lunch and dinner because they have fasted for 16 hours! Don't do that; if you

do, you risk experiencing weight gain instead of weight loss.
- There are of course initial side effects such as dizziness and nausea because the body is still adjusting to the new diet pattern.

HOW TO START WITH THE 16:8 INTERVAL?

First, you need to ascertain if you have a history of diseases such as diabetes and high blood pressure. If you are in this bracket (and if you are taking any medication), please consult your physician first before commencing. Never go through this IF method if you are trying to conceive, are breastfeeding, or pregnant/suspect you are pregnant.

Next is for you to choose a comfortable eating-window. Try the 16:8 IF once or twice in a week and see the effect it has on you. If you see that the side effects are ebbing away and your body is getting comfortable, you can increase the frequency to thrice a week, and so on until – if it is your preference – the 16:8 interval becomes a daily routine.

Once again, in IF, you are in control.

THE 20:4 INTERVAL

Are you ready for an even more challenging approach to losing weight? Then gear up for the 20:4 interval. Some people call this format the Warrior Diet because of the vibe – if you can only eat in a four-hour eating-window, then you are indeed a triumphant warrior. For instance, if you choose 12:00 noon to 4:00 in the afternoon as your eating-window, then you can only eat food during that time. Nothing more after that said period.

Imagine that!

Well, the way I have phrased everything may be a little intimidating, but according to Keto Concern, the 20:4 method isn't that bad. Read more for the details.

The Pros

- If you bring out the mathematician in you, in the 20 hours that you are fasting, you'll be asleep (ideally) for 8 hours. In our waking time, we only fast for 12 hours. That doesn't sound half as bad now, does it?
- You won't be completely void of nutrition during the 20 hours as you can drink non-calorie liquids like unsweetened tea.
- Do I hear savings? Because you will definitely be able to save with this diet! Imagine not eating for most of the day.
- Rules are not as strict as it may seem; people who are under this interval sometimes "snack very lightly" during the 20 hours. Experts say it's better to snack than to totally quit.
- Look at many Keto and Low Carb websites, and they will tell you that should other intervals not work for you, this one would. It's that effective.
- You can plan and enjoy what you will eat during the 4 hours window.

The Cons

- I wonder if any food lover has ever survived this scheme because it as though you must dislike eating to take this diet seriously. Barely eating for 20 hours seems like a very uphill climb.
- This is definitely a no-no for people who have medical conditions like diabetes as they need to maintain certain levels of blood sugar.

HOW TO START WITH THE 20:4 INTERVAL?

Well, a lot of people will only resort to this interval if the 16:8 didn't work out for them. If you are a food lover and the 16:8 method is working out just fine; no need to proceed to this "stage". If the need arises, proceed only if you are *very* comfortable with the 16:8 interval, otherwise your body might be pushed too hard, too soon.

Once ready, prepare your meals. A lot of people have one big meal AND continuous light snacks for 4 hours. Since this will be your ONLY meal, you might as well think about it carefully. Next is to prepare the drinks you'll bring with you.

Last but not least, remember to transition. Never go from hero to zero when it comes to any IF interval, especially this one. You cannot feast for 20 years and decide that you'll only eat on a 4-hour time-frame tomorrow.

WHAT ABOUT THE 12:12 THAT I HAVE HEARD OF?

Before we advance to the "easier" versions of intermittent fasting, let me first introduce you to the 12:12 method. Now, for many people, this isn't valid intermittent fasting because the idea of IF is to fast for longer hours and eat for less. With 12:12 approach, you get a 12-hour eating-window and a 12-hour fasting time. Still, I would like to include it in this paragraph because, in my opinion, this can be a springboard for those who want to go through the 16:8 interval and if necessary the 20:4. In 12:12, there will be few changes as you are actually already doing it – say you eat at 7 am and have dinner at 7 pm before going to sleep. The effort lies in making sure that there will be no super early morning meals, late night and midnight snacks. Also, you need to be strict to really not eat anything during the 12 hours. The best strategy is to cleanse your diet of empty calories and start preparing it for the healthier, fewer choices.

THE 5:2 INTERVAL

When I first heard of intermittent fasting and learned of the two previous methods, 16:8 and 20:4, I can't seem to "guess" what the 5:2 interval is. The numbers just don't add up to 24. They add up to 7 – the number of days in a week. With this, I became excited.

True enough when I did a little digging, I found out that in the 5:2 diet, you can eat WHATEVER you want for 5 days and eat barely for the other This seemed like an appealing way for me to lose weight because, to be honest, who doesn't want shed off extra pounds AND still get to eat cakes and pasta?!

Okay, so eating pretty much anything for 5 days is easy, but how do you fast for the two days? According to BBC Good Food, you need to cut back your "normal" caloric intake by 75%. That means that if your usual calorie intake is 2,000, then you can only have about 1000 calories for those two days when you are fasting (500 each day).

The Pros

- I'd say being able to eat whatever I like 5 days a week is a strong point. If you undergo the 16:8 or 20:4 method, you can't do that.
- Fewer restrictions because you don't have to exclude any food group such as carbs, salty foods, etc.
- Fast results - Experts say that with this diet, someone can lose 1 lb. in just one week!

The Cons

- The idea of eating anything might be misunderstood as "you can eat anything at whatever amount", which isn't

good because the diet suggests that you eat "normally" for 5 days
- More computations because you need to check on the caloric content of the food.

HOW TO START WITH THE 5:2 INTERVAL?

Take heart! You must be thinking: can I possibly go for two days with just 1000 calories in total? No worries because you actually CANNOT fast for two consecutive days. To start this 5:2 diet, you need to choose two days in a week when you'll fast, just make sure that there's at least ONE non-fasting day between them. The most common (according to blogs) is choosing Mondays and Thursdays.

Next step is to count your calories. Remember that you will need to maintain only 25% of whatever result you'll get. A woman with an active lifestyle who consumes 2,400 daily needs to only have 600 daily for the two days she chooses to fast. In the days when you'll fast, you can choose between eating 3 small meals or two slightly bigger ones. There are no restrictions on when you'll eat them.

And last but not that least, consider your health. When in doubt, always ask your physician, especially if you have eating disorders or conditions such as diabetes or are pregnant. Typically, bouts of hunger can be experienced, but dieters say they'll fade away especially if you keep busy. For the first times, you'll fast it'll be wise to have small snacks handy for the episodes when the hunger becomes intolerable.

THE 6:1 INTERVAL

You guessed it right! With a 6:1 interval, you can eat normally for 6 days and fast on one day. But when I say fast, I actually mean fast – for 24 hours! Even though in the 5:2 diet you're allowed to at least have 25% of the normal caloric intake, that's not the case with 6:1 where you'll have to fast entirely. If you're familiar with the band

Coldplay, you would find it interesting to note that their vocalist Chris Martin, is a huge fan of this diet. He says that he can sing and focus better by fasting for 24 hours.

The Pros

- Live the life! Eating anything six times a week is tantamount to not dieting at all!
- Again, no food group restrictions.

The Cons

- The craving for high-caloric food after 24 hours of fasting may be strong. Imagine fasting for one day and then eating 3 slices of pizza, 2 donuts, and drinking 1 bottle of sweetened soda after. That'll kind of defeat the purpose of living the healthy lifestyle which IF is promoting.
- There can be a significant lack of concentration and mood swings may happen on the day of fasting.
- The main, but somewhat hidden message of this diet to eat healthy for 6 days is ignored by many, as they choose to eat high-carb and high-salt foods because they are heaven to the taste buds.

HOW TO START THE 6:1 INTERVAL?

Consider the points of the 5:2 diet – choose the day you'll fast. Make it the day when you'll do nothing but relax, preferably Saturday or Sunday when you're off so that there is no need to focus. Next is to prepare your drinks because that's the only thing you're allowed to have on the day of fasting. Aside from water, you can have herbal and fruit tea as well as black tea. Just make sure that you don't have more than 3 cups of caffeinated drinks.

All of these intermittent fasting methods are effective; you only need to choose the type which will suit you best.

ASK YOURSELF:

How long are you able to fast in one sitting?
In what method do you see yourself succeeding?
What interval does your job allow you to have?

Reflect on these questions and then set out to read about other people's experience of the chosen interval.

If you are still unsure of what you want to do, just choose one Fasting Interval from above and try it out. You will then determine whether the interval is something for you. And if not, you can still switch. Testing is the name of the game.

4

WEIGHT LOSS AND INTERMITTENT FASTING

Here's the thing: there are countless diets around, and the proponents including those who have lost weight using them will state that "It's the best diet ever!" In fact, allow me to say that almost every year, a new diet technique will emerge, and people will "try them out" to see if the testimonials are correct or if they're just a scam.

While you may go wrong with other diets because restrict you from eating certain food groups IF is different as you may have already noticed. But why exactly is intermittent fasting better than doing diets?

THE BENEFITS OF INTERMITTENT FASTING

- First and foremost, fasting is an age-old way to lose weight. Even our grandparents and great grandparents have – at least once in their life – tried fasting. YOU are fasting each time you stop eating after dinner and go to sleep. In other words, you don't need to "experiment" with IF – you only have to modify it in such a way that its weight-losing potential can be maximized.

- When a diet asks you to count the calories that's because it wants you to eat less than you normally do, that's because it wants you to burn calories. That's also the main idea in IF, especially in the 16:8 and 20:4 interval – fast more and feast less. The best part is you DON'T need to count the calories unless you're going for the 5:2 diet.
- No one is telling you what to eat. Let's admit it – many diet systems around WILL tell you to eat this, have this meal plan, buy this food, and blend this concoction. IF won't require you to do anything other than *choose when to eat*. And you have so much control over that! With several options, you can ponder on what IF is best for you and your lifestyle.
- Intermittent fasting is so versatile. Aside from the control, let's not forget that IF can be partnered with other diet systems which you find effective for you. For instance, many people do intermittent fasting WHILE doing the low-carb diet; that's why we have numerous Facebook groups for Low-Carb Intermittent Fasting. Another popular diet commonly partnered with IF is a ketogenic diet, where you are encouraged to eat more healthy fats.
- Boosting metabolism? Intermittent fasting is also anchored to that! Other diet systems which tell you that you can lose weight with them, because they boost the metabolism may not be lying, but IF can also do that. The reason why we're cutting back on the eating window is because we "encourage" our body to metabolize the distributed, hard-earned fats.
- And lastly, experts in Men's Journal said that "there are really no downsides to intermittent fasting". The only question would be how effective it's going to be after you've made it your lifestyle.

THERE IS NO YO-YO EFFECT BECAUSE IF IS A LIFESTYLE

This is actually another benefit of IF, but since the yo-yo effect is common to other diet systems, I want a separate section to explain this. The yo-yo effect is when you cycle between losing weight and gaining weight. In other words, after trying a diet (say for 2 months) you lose weight, but after some time, you also gain weight; going up and down, sort of like a yo-yo.

WHY DOES THIS HAPPEN?

To put it simply other methods are hard to maintain. Hence people tend to "take a break" – that's when they experience the yo-yo effect. Let's say your diet requires you to take in fruit and vegetable smoothies for whatever number of days in a week. Making a smoothie is sometimes inconvenient, and if you have a busy lifestyle, you might not be able to catch up. Other systems are also expensive, so when the budget becomes tight, you need to cut back.

Since intermittent fasting is a lifestyle, there's no yo-yo effect.

IF is fairly easy so there's really no need to take a break. It will take some time getting used to, but quitting is not necessary. When the hunger becomes unbearable IF allows you to have a quick small snack. It's also very lenient when it comes to liquid consumption. The 16:8 interval even has a level of normalcy to it except for the skipping breakfast part.

5

BEGINNER MISTAKES ON INTERMITTENT FASTING

Do you remember the first time you tried to drive a car? Didn't you make A LOT of mistakes? That's the way it always is when it comes to learning a new skill. Doing intermittent fasting is no different. While trying to follow all the rules, remember that it's normal to catch yourself making several errors. The important thing is not the error, but that you catch yourself. Don't lose the will to reset the diet. Even experts agree that committing the errors is a part of the learning curve. Below are some of the most common mistakes one can make when starting out with IF.

STILL EATING THE WRONG FOODS ALL THE TIME

Do you know that the feeling of deprivation is very powerful? When you have gone through a week of not holding your phone, you most probably will not let go of it the minute you have it in your hands. When you are fasting, you feel the same deprivation; and because you are deprived your cravings will revolve around delicious, unhealthy foods such as candies, shakes, pasta and salted crackers.

Think about it – the times you are eating are limited, so you have to make the most of it. Nourish your system with healthy amounts of fats, fiber, carbs, protein, vitamins and minerals.

How can you avoid the mistake of eating the wrong foods? Simple. Each time you eat, ask yourself if the foods you are taking are worth wasting all your efforts for. Believe me when I say that healthy food doesn't have to taste bad – with correct combinations they can actually be satisfying. My advice is to prepare a meal plan which will outline your food for the whole week. Under the 16:8 approach, what will be your lunch and dinner? What snacks can you prepare?

YOU START TOO AMBITIOUS AND GIVE UP TOO FAST

When I first started with intermittent fasting, I began with the 16:8 method RIGHT AWAY. As in no preparation whatsoever. My body – and my mind – was admittedly shocked. The result? I gave up the diet as fast as I started it.

My personal advice to you is this: whatever interval you choose, prepare your mind and body. Clear your pantry from the empty-calorie food. Try a healthy meal here and there. Feel the effect of fasting. Consider modifying the timeframe. If you feel hungry have a little snack – just don't give up altogether.

Intermittent fasting is a lifestyle so you can't hurry it up. The crucial part is the beginning, so tread carefully. It's better to start out slow than rush along and fail.

THE FEAR OF FEELING HUNGRY BECOMES TOO STRONG

If you have a job that keeps you fed, chances are you're not afraid to be hungry; at least not in the sense that you won't be able to buy food. Well, that's not the fear we are talking about here. As an employed or supported individual, you tend to be so used to eating the complete set of meals with some snacks in between. What do you think will happen when you begin intermittent fasting? Let me tell you: there will be a point in practicing IF when you'd fear hunger. You will fear that being hungry will ruin your good start. You will be scared that hunger can drive you to eat unhealthy foods. You worry that you become too hungry too fast even when your eating-window just ended. All these will lead you to constantly fear that hunger and the power of temptation sets in. That imaginary hunger becomes real.

To avoid this, keep yourself busy. If there's something you can do, do it now so there will be no room for worrying about the hunger that maybe isn't even there. If the urge to eat becomes intolerable, get your snack or liquid ready. Give yourself a break. Being hungry is natural and for a beginner, expected.

BEING OBSESSED WITH THE CLOCK - WHEN CAN I BINGE?

IF is anchored in the idea of eating only when it's time. I myself even had the notion that the clock will dictate when my eating-window will begin and when it ends. Here's a secret – that's not entirely correct. This article at Two Meal Day says that the reason why the timeframes are created is so that we will be in tune with our body. Since we are fasting, we will be able to feel our system without the distraction of eating. Real hunger, according to the same article, is something that occurs once every 16 to 24 hours – not every 4!

When you obsess over "Is it time to eat yet?" or "Do I still have time to eat this?" then you are not feeling your body – you're feeling the clock. The best way to improve the situation is to set an alarm and let it be. Eventually, you will notice that the alarm is not necessary anymore because your body will alert you if it needs nourishment.

CHOOSING THE WRONG INTERVAL

For all you know, the interval of your choice will be your dietary lifestyle forever. For this reason, you must choose the timeframe carefully. The sad truth about any diet is you can't measure your compatibility with it ahead of time; you need to try it out first before you can be certain. Intermittent fasting is no exception.

Don't worry too much though, because there are guidelines that you can follow to NOT second guess the interval for you.

Choose the 16:8 if:

- You can skip one meal (probably breakfast) WITHOUT eating more than normal for the other two meals.
- If you are a beginner and want to try intermittent fasting to lose weight.
- You have a career that needs constant nourishment throughout the day.

Choose the 20:4 if:

- You have gone through 16:8 successfully for at least months without any problem.
- The 16:8 method didn't work the way you wanted it to work for you, and you feel that there's a need to "escalate" things a little bit.
- You're a person who has a career that's not too physically active.

Choose the 5:2 if:

- You can only tolerate fasting once in a while.
- You can control what you eat even when you are not fasting – as there's a tendency to binge on unhealthy foods in the 5 days you can eat.
- The number of calories you need in your lifestyle is naturally low.

Choose 6:1 if:

- You can tolerate eating nothing for ONE FULL DAY.
- You can remind yourself consistently that while you are not fasting for the other 6 days, healthy food selection is still the best.
- You have at least one day when the only thing you'll do is relax and fast.

The advice still stands: test the waters first before choosing an interval. There's no need to hop onto the wagon right away.

EATING TOO MUCH

Eating too much when the time to eat arrives is common at the beginning of intermittent fasting. The hunger is so palpable because our body is still trying to grasp the new routine. The point in IF is to consume fewer calories and burn more, so if you'll compensate then the whole point is ruined.

For you to avoid this error, you need to know your portions and eat slowly. When you eat slowly, you're giving your body enough time to process the ingested food. Soon enough you'll feel satiated, and there'll be no need to eat anymore. On the other side, if you binge eat fast, you won't feel that your body has already had enough food and you will believe you need more.

EATING TOO LITTLE

The opposite of binge eating is restricting yourself during the eating window. In fear of binge eating, someone starting with the intermittent fasting would still take in fewer calories than normal. This isn't good; our body is like a machine that needs fuel in the form of food. During the eating-window think of how you would commonly eat at the time – make healthier food choices but DON'T calorie-restrict anymore because you've already done that while you were in the fasting state.

FORGETTING TO DRINK

Drinking water is important not only because you don't want to become dehydrated but because it will help you flush out toxin breakdowns while you are in the fasting state. Moreover, the more you drink water, the less likely you'll feel the hunger. Always bring a jug of water with you wherever you go. When you have time, consider taking in other non-calorie drinks such as unsweetened teas.

On a final note for this section, please understand that committing a mistake is okay. It's normal and will definitely happen at the beginning of your IF journey. Don't be discouraged when you make blunders.

6

HOW TO MOTIVATE YOURSELF

Isn't losing weight enough of a motivation to continue intermittent fasting? The ugly truth is, it isn't. In fact, when the climb becomes too steep, you will even consider throwing in the white towel and make excuses such as "I'll just love my body the way it is." Don't get me wrong – loving your body just the way it is, is beautiful. However, if you don't really feel like loving it now and are just using the adage to excuse yourself from the efforts, try again.

In this chapter, I will list things that can motivate you to keep going.

REMIND YOURSELF OF WHY YOU STARTED

As the infamous saying goes, when you're about to give up think of why you wanted to begin in the first place. Why did you start IF? Is it not to lose weight and feel good? Is it not to become healthier that you may enjoy life more for longer? Are you giving up on all these goals just because the beginning is too difficult?

Of course not.

So, remind yourself by making a vision board, by buying a promise ring, or by hanging that beautiful dress by your bedroom door. Whatever helps you to persevere, do it because most of the time the hardest part of any journey is just the beginning.

PROGRESS IS THE BEST MOTIVATOR – SO DON'T STOP UNTIL YOU WEIGH AT LEAST 1 POUND LESS!

Once you've crossed the hurdle of beginning IF, it's time to motivate yourself even further by tracking your progress. To do this, keep a notepad by your table and record your weight weekly. If you have the time, you might as well record the foods you ate for one whole week! You'll be surprised to know that you can EAT healthily without being too grumpy about it. In my opinion, that in itself is already an achievement.

Aside from recording the figures, why don't you take a picture weekly while wearing a shirt that fits just about right for you? Over the weeks, wear the same shirt and watch as it becomes bigger for you.

Or my favorite way to track progress is to watch how my used-to-be small dress fits me after weeks of doing intermittent fasting.

How about you? Can you think of another way to track your progress? Because believe me when I say that once you see an improvement, stopping is next to impossible. You will want more of that improvement.

REWARD YOURSELF

Oooh! Rewards. Don't you think it's high time for you to reward yourself after such efforts? Not with food, preferably, but something you really want to have or somewhere you want to go to.

Here are some of the milestones which you can consider as an achievement (and therefore be the reason for the rewards)

- Being able to finish a day of intermittent fasting

- Knowing that for one full day, you didn't eat anything unhealthy like junk foods
- Strictly going through IF for one whole week
- Losing that first pound
- Realizing that you're now one size smaller!

Please note that your achievement doesn't have to be grand just as your rewards don't have to be expensive. The following can be your reward:

- Watching a film
- Buying a book or anything small you'd like to have
- Having a spa day
- Going out with friends on a movie night
- Having a small piece of chocolate

Rewards help you tamper the feeling of deprivation, so go on, reward yourself.

REMOVE NEGATIVE PEOPLE OUT OF YOUR LIFE

I'll make it short and simple, if someone at home or in your office is discouraging you from continuing IF, keep them out of your IF routine. I'm not saying that you literally have to stop being friends with them – just that you have to be firm in saying that they have no say where your weight loss goal is concerned. When they say something bad, let the words in one ear and out the other. Don't argue. Just ignore them. They can't see nor feel the progress in your body – you can. The only person who can stop you from doing IF is yourself.

BE ACCOUNTABLE

Whatever you do, it's your choice. That's what you need to keep reminding yourself. You can't blame intermittent fasting because it's too hard; you can't say it's your family's fault for not being supportive and you definitely shouldn't let your schedule stop you. Everything is on you. I'm not saying this to make you feel bad for not trying hard enough, but because the core of intermittent fasting is to let the individual stay in control. If you let the timeframes, your schedule, and other people manipulate you into stopping, then you are not entirely in control.

Remember: it's your body and therefore your responsibility.

REMIND YOURSELF OF WHAT WILL HAPPEN IF YOU DON'T ACT NOW

I know all about delaying tactics – they are addictive. You keep on saying you'll start tomorrow, or next week, or next month, but that time NEVER COMES. The best time to start is NOW. Again, when I say start, I'm not referring to the actual fast, but the preparation.

Take it one day at a time.

For the first week, clear out your fridge of sodas and remove all the junk foods in your dining area. Replace it with healthy alternatives such as nuts, fruits, and teas. On the second week, try fasting during breakfast, dinner or lunch. There are many more things you can do to START intermittent fasting now, so don't delay because if you do, you're wasting precious time.

Who knows, if you start now maybe you'll be able to see the results next month? More than external motivation, you need an inner boost to follow through with intermittent fasting.

7

INTERMITTENT FASTING IS NOT FOR EVERYONE

The sad fact is this: intermittent fasting is not for everyone. If you're a fairly healthy individual who wants to be more fit and have more energy, intermittent fasting can work wonders for you. However, other people won't be able to tolerate systematic fasting.

IF is not suitable for people with diabetes as most of them need insulin shots – remember that intermittent fasting will lower insulin levels. It's also not recommended for people taking blood thinners.

Women who are pregnant or are planning to conceive must not undergo IF; likewise when a mother is breastfeeding. People under 18 should not resort to intermittent fasting. Should the BMI be 18.5 or lower, never consider IF, also if you have eating disorders. If you have a medical condition, talk to your doctor first before fasting.

Intermittent Fasting Dos

- Determine if you're okay to fast (consider the abovementioned conditions)
- Think carefully about your schedule. When can you fast? What time of the day or day of the week is best for you? This is needed so that you can fit IF into your lifestyle.

- Prepare your mind and body (as well as your pantry and fridge)
- Take your vitamins – due to fasting and the food choices, the vitamins in your body might need to be replenished. Choose vitamins in liquid form so that you can still take it during times when you are fasting.
- Do IF with friends because it's fun that way and more motivating.
- Take it easy when breaking your fast. When your eating-window starts, don't gorge on high carb, high-fat meal! Take it easy. Have a salad and something with high protein.

Intermittent Fasting Dont's

- Do hardcore workouts when fasting. That's pushing your body too much.
- Ignore your body when it's telling you something. If you can't focus, feel sick, and are really, really hungry, stop fasting. Have a snack or a full meal if you must. Remember, one step at a time. If there's a need to stop, then stop fasting.
- Stress. Don't stress yourself, especially when fasting.
- Drink unsweetened sodas and juice UNLESS you're in your eating window. In fact, if you can, don't take sweetened drinks at all.

To put it simply, intermittent fasting is good for anyone without any medical condition that can make it dangerous for them to fast. I hope for sure that you are included in the "go" bracket because the effects of IF are phenomenal and I want you to experience them. In the next chapter, we will be discussing the Frequently Asked Questions.

8

FREQUENTLY ASKED QUESTIONS

In this final chapter, I'd like to address your most frequently asked questions. Please don't get frustrated that some of the answers here are not exact because that's just really the case. As we have reiterated again and again, IF depends vastly on the individual, so the effects are also unique for the person doing the fast.

HOW LONG DOES IT TAKE TO SEE ANY EFFECTS?

According to LifeHack.org, in intermittent fasting, you can lose as much as 2-3 pounds in a week depending on how long you fast and what you eat when your eating-window is up. The 2-3 pounds in a week is more commonly seen on the 16:8 and 20:4 interval. If your result is less than that, it's okay.

So, to answer the original question, you can see the results in as little as one week.

WHAT IS THE BEST TIME TO FAST?

The best way to fast is completely dependent on your body, your preference, or your lifestyle. If you can skip breakfast (or just one meal for that matter), the 16:8 method might just be right for you. For the 20:4 diet, you might need to choose an eating-window that will keep you focused while working. Try 12:00 pm to 4:00 pm because that's the bulk of where the work is if you're working a 9 am to 5 pm job. With a 5:2 interval, consider what we've mentioned earlier – Mondays and Thursdays – as the fasting days because there are at least 2 non-fasting days between them. Of course, with 6:1, I suggest you choose Saturday or Sunday because that's your most relaxed days.

WHAT SHOULD I EAT WHEN I AM NOT FASTING?

When not fasting, you need to replenish your energy and prepare it for the activities of the day and the incoming fast. For this reason, I have prepared a list which you can use as a reference on the foods to eat and liquids to drink.

- Highly satiating foods such as avocado. Even though avocado is high in calories, it's very satisfying. Half of this fruit can make you feel full for hours longer than if you won't eat it.
- Fish. Since we need fats and proteins in healthy proportion, go with fish. Not only is it good for breaking the fast but you can also prepare it in several ways.
- Fibrous greens. Vegetables are rich in vitamins and minerals that we won't get from other sources. Not only that but eating healthy portions of these will cleanse your colon and make certain that it is in a top condition to release waste. If you can, consider taking in probiotics because they do wonders for the digestive system as well.
- Whole grains are a great source of protein and fiber, and they keep you feel just as much satiated as white bread, and white rice do. They may be a little pricey, but since you are technically fasting, perhaps they will be more affordable.

- Eggs because of its richness in protein.
- Potatoes as a source of carbohydrates; it's also highly satiating. NOTE: Potato crackers and fries don't count.
- Nuts which are great as snacks and are rich in good fats.
- Water and non-caloric drinks.

When you dig in a little, you'll know that there are a lot of good foods around the corner, so bring out your trusty mobile phones and search for recipes!

IS INTERMITTENT FASTING SUITABLE FOR DAILY LIFE?

Definitely! As I mentioned earlier, you are already fasting every day! With intermittent fasting, we will just modify it a little bit and toughen it up to maximize the calorie-burning capacity of the body. There are of course times when you need to stop fasting because of strenuous activities or because you are sick but other than that, daily fasting is okay especially if you're taking it slowly.

HOW LONG CAN I FAST SAFELY?

Well, it really depends on you. Hardcore intermittent fasting enthusiasts have already made it their lifestyle to fast with the interval of their choice. Still, since control is the name of the game, you can modify the frequency depending on your need and capacity. As a beginner, you can start out small by say doing a 16:8 interval one week in a month, then down to every other week until eventually, you can do it every day in your life with a few cheat days in between.

Just remember the golden rule: listen to your body. If it needs nourishment, then break the rules and eat.

HOW DO I DEAL WITH HUNGER DURING FASTING?

The first question is, are you really hungry or you're just thinking about food? If you're just thinking about food, keep yourself busy or have a fun distraction for a few minutes until the obsession to eat fades away. If your body is telling you that you are indeed hungry, try to drink water or tasty, no-calorie drinks like unsweetened herbal teas. Your last resort is to eat, and when you do, you won't gorge on junk foods. Rather, you must choose foods with a low-glycemic index or those foods that have the least effect to your blood sugar level. Examples of these foods with low GI are beans and lentils.

CAN I EXERCISE WHILE FASTING?

The short answer to this question is YES, but I'd much rather give you the long answer. You can exercise while fasting but make sure that it's short and not that exertive. According to this article, after more than a week of intermittent fasting, their energy is significantly boosted. Don't forget that walking and jogging are considered workouts, so you don't have an excuse to not exercise.

The next question now is this: do I exercise before I eat or after I have eaten? This still depends on you, but my suggestion is to do it *before* you eat because there's a chance that you will feel hungry after exercising. That way, you will feel extremely satisfied when eating. Now, if you work out after you have eaten a meal, you might feel the hunger again and be encouraged to eat more than what's enough.

Again, exercising is good but not when your body is craving rest and sleep. What workout can you do that won't ruin your fasting?

AFTERWORD

Alright!

That one was a tough; informative ride wasn't it? First of all, congratulations on reading the entire book. I don't know how long it took you to read everything from the introduction to this part, but it doesn't matter. For all I know, you started with IF when you read about the different intervals.

Sincerely, I hope that you learned a lot from this book. Before we formally end this journey, I would like to give you a timeframe of how you can proceed with intermittent fasting.

Starting now (yes, as in now), refrain from eating unhealthy foods such as store-bought soda, junk foods, donuts with sugar content as high as the clouds, and others. There's no harm in healthy choices, right? Do it for about a week and see the changes in your mood and energy. For the second week (even little by little) re-arrange your kitchen and dining area in such a way that the only foods allowed are the healthy ones. You can still have a few junk foods and chocolates here and there but be sure to only consume them once in a while. For the third week, choose an interval for you. You can read more from other blogs and other websites. Try it out and see how your body will react. At this point, since you are already eating healthily, your

AFTERWORD

system won't be shocked at the lowered calorie intake. When you notice that you can give it a go, begin with the intermittent fasting of your choice. Remember that mistakes are common, and that hunger may often be felt. BREAK the fast if your body tells you to do so.

The above example is just a simple timeline; of course, you can come up with your own scheme. The crucial part is the beginning so, start now while you can clearly remember that intermittent fasting offers a lot of benefits for your mind and body.

Once you have successfully incorporated IF into your life (say for a few months), try to partner it with other healthy diet methods such as the fast-emerging low carbs diet. You can also look into the paleo diet and ketogenic diet. Intermittent fasting is so versatile that you don't have to worry about its compatibility with other methods.

Last but not least I would like you to pat yourself on the back. The fact that you have finished reading this book says a lot about your determination. Don't let outside factors crush that perseverance.

If you liked this book, please let others know by submitting a review. Should you have any comments and suggestions, my line is open all the time. You can contact me at: Justine.young.books@gmail.com.

Intermittent fasting is a way of life, so let it evolve together with you. All the best and more power!

Justine Young

LAST WORDS

Thank you again for reading this book!

I hope this book was able to help and inspire you to start a new way of living. I am certain the information provided in this book

Finally, if you enjoyed this book, then I'd like to ask you a favor, would you be kind enough to leave a review for this book on Amazon? It'd be greatly appreciated!

Thank you and good luck!

BONUS

You want to get results faster? Why not give your Intermittent Fasting Journey a little head start?

Download your free copy of 22 Intermittent Fasting secret tips and tricks here: >> http://bit.ly/22tricks

REFERENCES

https://www.healthline.com/nutrition/16-8-intermittent-fasting#right-for-you
https://www.bbcgoodfood.com/howto/guide/what-52-diet
https://www.telegraph.co.uk/food-and-drink/news/what-is-the-61-diet/
https://www.nowtolove.co.nz/health/body/the-new-61-diet-23755
https://www.mindbodygreen.com/articles/why-intermittent-fasting-is-the-best-thing-to-ever-happen-to-your-metabolism
https://www.orangefit.nl/en/fit-blog/lifestyle/how-to-stop-the-yoyo-effect
https://michaelkummer.com/health/intermittent-fasting-benefits/
https://2mealday.com/article/top-5-intermittent-fasting-mistakes/
https://whatsgood.vitaminshoppe.com/intermittent-fasting-mistakes/
https://www.bornfitness.com/intermittent-fasting/
https://www.livestrong.com/slideshow/1008373-master-fast-dos-donts/?slide=13
https://superfastdiet.com/is-intermittent-fasting-for-everyone/
https://sheroes.com/articles/intermittent-fasting/NzE0NQ==

REFERENCES

https://www.lifehack.org/articles/lifestyle/intermittent-fasting-the-ultimate-weight-loss-hack.html
https://greatist.com/eat/what-to-eat-on-an-intermittent-fasting-diet
https://perfectketo.com/how-often-can-you-do-intermittent-fasting/
https://www.dummies.com/health/nutrition/weight-loss/9-ways-to-stave-off-hunger-when-fasting/#slide-9

© Copyright 2019 by Kok Yuan Tang - All rights reserved.

This document is geared towards providing exact and reliable information in regards to the topic and issue covered. The publication is sold with the idea that the publisher is not required to render accounting, officially permitted, or otherwise, qualified services. If advice is necessary, legal or professional, a practiced individual in the profession should be ordered. - From a Declaration of Principles which was accepted and approved equally by a Committee of the American Bar Association and a Committee of Publishers and Associations. In no way is it legal to reproduce, duplicate, or transmit any part of this document in either electronic means or in printed format. Recording of this publication is strictly prohibited and any storage of this document is not allowed unless with written permission from the publisher. All rights reserved. The information provided herein is stated to be truthful and consistent, in that any liability, in terms of inattention or otherwise, by any usage or abuse of any policies, processes, or directions contained within is the solitary and utter responsibility of the recipient reader. Under no circumstances will any legal responsibility or blame be held against the publisher for any reparation, damages, or monetary loss due to the information herein, either directly or indirectly. Respective authors own all copyrights not held by the publisher. The information herein is offered for informational purposes solely, and is universal as so. The presentation of the information is without contract or any type of guarantee assurance. The trademarks that are used are without any consent, and the publication of the trademark is without permission or backing by the trademark owner. All trademarks and brands within this book are for clarifying purposes only and are the owned by the owners themselves, not affiliated with this document.

Made in the USA
Monee, IL
04 November 2022